Understanding
Acupuncture

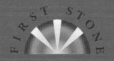

FIRST STONE

Contents

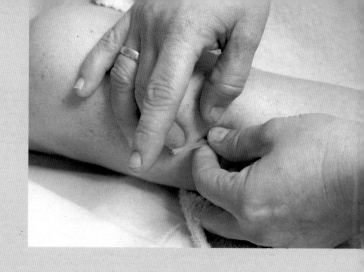

1

Introducing Acupuncture

Acupuncture is a system of medicine that aims to restore and maintain health by the insertion of fine needles into specific points on the body.

Needling these points (i.e. placing needles into the skin at specific points – see picture on left) stimulates the body to 'rebalance' itself, encouraging homoeostasis (maintaining our internal systems in a state of equilibrium) by activating our own self-healing powers.

ORIGINS

Acupuncture forms a part of Traditional Chinese Medicine (TCM), an ancient form of healing that developed over several thousands of years,

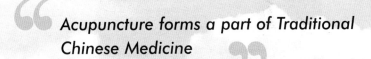

Acupuncture forms a part of Traditional Chinese Medicine

mostly in China, but also in Japan and other parts of the Far East (see Chapter Two).

WHO CAN IT HELP?

In the West, acupuncture is associated with pain relief and addiction problems, although most people are also aware that the Chinese use acupuncture as a form of anaesthetic.

In fact, there are few health problems that acupuncture has not been used to treat. The World Health Organisation (WHO) has compiled a list of diseases and conditions for which it considers treatment with acupuncture to be appropriate. On this list are:

• **Respiratory problems:**
  Bronchitis, bronchial asthma, acute sinusitis, acute rhinitis,

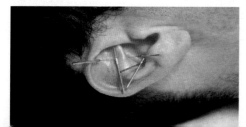

There are several acu-points in the ear that can be used in the treatment of addiction.

common cold, and acute tonsillitis.

- **Gastrointestinal problems:** Diarrhoea, constipation, hiccups, gastritis, gastric hyperacidity, chronic duodenal ulcer, dysentery, acute bacillary dysentery, paralytic ileus, and spasms of oesophagus and cardia.
- **Mouth problems:** Toothache, post-extraction pain, gingivitis, acute and chronic pharyngitis.
- **Eye problems:** Acute conjunctivitis, central

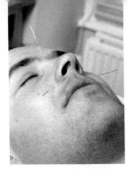

Acupuncture can also be used to treat specific problems, such as acute sinusitis.

retinitis, childhood myopia, and cataracts.

- **Neurological and musculoskeletal disorders:** Headache, migraine, facial neuralgia, facial palsy, muscle weakness following a stroke, problems of the peripheral nervous system, problems resulting

7

from polio, Ménière's disease, neurogenic bladder dysfunction, nocturnal enuresis, neuralgia in the rib area, cervicobrachial syndrome, frozen shoulder, tennis elbow, sciatica, low-back pain, and osteoarthritis.

Acupuncture has also been used to treat many other problems, as wide-ranging as gynaecological conditions, problems arising from pregnancy and childbirth, addictions, impotence, insomnia, schizophrenia, varicose veins, vertigo, eczema, colitis, infectious hepatitis and shingles.

It has been claimed that acupuncture can 'usually treat every condition, but not cure every case', which is perhaps as much as any treatment can realistically aim for.

RESEARCH

In the past 30 years, more than 500 randomised, controlled trials have been undertaken in the West to investigate acupuncture – primarily in the treatment of pain, but also other health problems.

In 1997, after sifting through this evidence, the National Institute of Health's Consensus Development Panel on Acupuncture, concluded that needle acupuncture is an effective treatment for:

- Post-operative and chemotherapy nausea and vomiting, and most probably, pregnancy-related nausea.
- Post-operative dental pain, menstrual cramps, tennis elbow and fibromyalgia, suggesting that acupuncture may have a more general effect on pain.

The fact that there is not more evidence in favour of the use of acupuncture is largely to do with the problems scientists have had in designing clinical trials – in particular, finding a suitable placebo control. There have been concerns expressed that needling anywhere in the body – at both real acupuncture sites or at non-acupuncture sites – may have physiological consequences that go beyond the effects scientists expect from an inert sham control such as those used in drug trials.

9

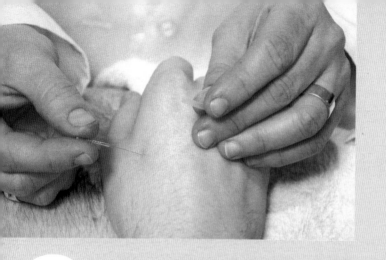

2

A Brief History

There is a legend that, some 7,000 years ago, Chinese physicians observed that soldiers wounded by arrows sometimes recovered from illnesses, unrelated to their injuries, that had afflicted them for many years.

From this observation acupuncture has developed, based on the principle that diseases can be treated by penetrating the skin at particular points. Presumably, the physicians quickly realised that the size of the wound did not matter, only its location.

The truth of this story is unknown, but it illustrates the importance of detailed observation in acupuncture. Certainly, it was through observation that Chinese physicians identified which points on the skin affected and controlled specific organs. They went on to show that, by penetrating these points with needles, a wide range of diseases could be cured.

It is generally believed that the first needles were made of stone, and stone needles have been found in ancient tombs in Inner Mongolia dating from 2,500 BC. Wood, bone and ceramic needles were also used. Bronze needles became popular around 3,000 years ago, during the Chang dynasty. Today, however, needles are made of stainless steel.

Different metals were thought to have different effects, and the Chinese found that using a gold needle for example, would stimulate; whereas silver would sedate. Although in Japan this approach is still taken, in China it fell into disuse as physicians focused on the way needles were applied in order to produce a given effect.

EARLY WRITINGS

Early writings on Chinese medicine date back more than 2,000 years, when a collection of 34 books was published under the title *Huang Di Nei Jing* (*The Yellow Emperor's Classic of Internal Medicine*).

This collection took hundreds of years to complete and still forms the basis of Traditional Chinese Medicine today (see Chapter Three). The earliest surviving work devoted exclusively to acupuncture is probably *A Classic of Acupuncture and Moxibustion*, written by Huang Fu Mi, published in 249AD. In it, the system of meridians and acupuncture points are described, along with their properties and indications.

In the Tang dynasty (618-907 AD) medical academies were established. In 1026, the *Classic of the Bronze Man* was published, which became a standard work, offering an illustrated guide to points, as shown on two life-size bronze acupuncture figures.

POPULARITY

The use of acupuncture spread to other Far Eastern countries during the 7th century, and continued to flourish throughout the region well into the 20th century. In the late 19th and early 20th Century, however, there was a decline in its popularity, as Western medicine was introduced to China. In 1929, the Kuomintang Government tried to ban all forms of traditional medicine.

This attempt failed. When the People's Republic of China was created in 1949, interest in acupuncture resurfaced, particularly in combination with Western medicine.

The Government embarked on a programme of modernisation, and initiated research to investigate the efficacy of Traditional Chinese Medicine. On the basis of its findings, traditional and modern medicine were accorded equal status under the Republic.

During the Cultural Revolution (1966-1976) Chinese medicine was often the only form of medicine available due to the persecution of surgeons and doctors practising Western medicine. Today, the two co-exist, giving patients a choice of both Western or Traditional Chinese Medicine approaches.

WESTERN ACUPUNCTURE

Acupuncture was introduced to the West during the 19th century, by Jesuit missionaries who had travelled to China and the Far East.

There are several recorded uses of acupuncture both in

France and Britain during this time. In 1929; Dr. Soulie de Morant published *L'Acupuncture Chinoise,* which he used as a text to teach traditional acupuncture to French doctors.

However, it was not until the 1950s and 1960s that the technique began to be taken seriously in Britain. Schools were established and regulatory organisations were set up. Training and regulation have continued to improve since, making acupuncture in the UK today an increasingly professional system.

TRADITIONAL AND MODERN

Acupuncture has now grown in popularity, to the extent that some medical doctors and physiotherapists use it as an adjunct to Western medicine. There are short training courses specially designed for them.

The acupuncture described in this book takes at least three years' full-time study to learn, and, while the focus is on traditional diagnosis and treatment, students also study Western medicine appropriate to the practise of acupuncture.

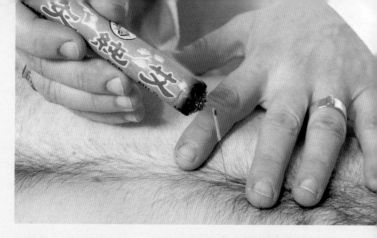

3

The Principles of Traditional Chinese Medicine

To understand acupuncture we must first understand the philosophical ideas that underpin it. Acupuncture forms a part of Traditional Chinese Medicine (TCM). TCM is an autonomous system of thought and practice quite unlike anything we are used to in the West.

HOLISTIC PRINCIPLES

Chinese medicine differs from conventional Western medicine in many significant ways. For example, TCM sees the 'spirit' as an important factor in overall health, and aspects that the Western world views as important (such as the nervous and endocrine systems) are not a part of Chinese medical theory.

The Western physician starts with a symptom, then searches for the underlying mechanism or cause of a specific disease. While the disease may affect various parts of the body, it is perceived as a relatively well-defined, self-contained phenomenon. The attention of the Chinese physician, in contrast, is on the patient as an individual. The patient's symptoms are set in the context of a complete physiological and psychological profile.

The information the Chinese physician gleans from his diagnostic techniques is woven together to form what the Chinese call a 'pattern of disharmony', describing a state of 'imbalance' in the patient's body.

PREVENTION

In Western medicine, the emphasis on prevention, as opposed to cure, has risen dramatically. However, prevention has been standard practice in TCM for millennia.

In the past, acupuncturists in China were paid by their patients to maintain their health. If someone fell ill, the acupuncturist was expected to treat them for free. As this passage from an ancient Chinese medical text (the *Nei Jing*) argues, "When medicinal therapy is initiated only after someone has fallen ill, when there is an attempt to restore order only after unrest has broken out, it is as though someone has waited to dig a well until he is already weak from thirst, or as if someone begins to forge a spear when the battle is already under way. Is this not too late?"

INDIVIDUALITY

While two patients presenting with identical symptoms may, in Western medicine, receive the same diagnosis and treatment, the same two patients may receive very different diagnoses and treatments from a Chinese physician.

This is because Chinese medicine seeks to understand how the symptoms fit into the patient's entire being and behaviour. But as Ted Kapchuk, an expert in Oriental medicine, has said, "The perceptions of the two traditions reflect two different worlds, but both can affect and often heal human beings regardless of their cultural affiliation".

HEAVEN AND EARTH

The Chinese believe that man lives between Heaven and Earth, two poles representing creativity and receptiveness, and givers of air (Heaven) and food (Earth). The energies and influences of Heaven and Earth combine in us to provide the energy necessary for life. This meeting of Heaven and Earth within a person must be kept in harmony and balance. Each of our internal organs has a particular function in this process, and must also work in harmony with the other organs. It is a finely-tuned system, so a problem with one organ will also affect the whole.

THE TAO (OR DAO)

The Tao is the 'path' or the 'way'– the way we do things or the way the universe works.

Living in harmony with the Tao is, for the Chinese, the essence of good health. Wisdom and knowledge come from attuning oneself ever more finely to the Tao.

To achieve this goal, balance is essential – balancing times of excitement with times of quiet reflection, balancing expenditure of energy with adequate nourishment, and so on. In Chinese terms, this means balancing the Yin and Yang aspects of life. If Yin and Yang become unbalanced (e.g. too much work and not enough rest), ill-health can result.

YIN AND YANG

The original meaning of the word 'Yin' was 'the shady side of the slope or the north bank of a river', while 'Yang' meant 'the sunny side of a slope or the south bank of a river'. These meanings have been expanded to describe the delicate balance of dark (Yin) and light (Yang). Yin/Yang expresses a system of relationships, patterns and functions, and the fundamental duality that exists in nature. This balance embraces all opposites – female and male, cold and hot, passivity and activity, in-breath and out-breath, sleeping and waking.

In Chinese medicine, Yin/Yang is used to describe and distinguish patterns of

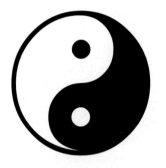

The Tai Ji symbol illustrates the balance between Yin and Yang, showing that the two are in a dynamic state of balance and that one cannot exist without the other.

disharmony. Reflection suggests Yin, action Yang; fast, sudden onset suggests Yang, slow and lingering conditions are Yin; under-activity is Yin, over-activity, Yang.

The Chinese believe that nothing is ever entirely Yin or Yang, that everything has within it the possibility of changing into its opposite. This idea is best illustrated by the well-known Tai Ji symbol. The dark and light are in balance and the small circles of white and black represent this idea that nothing is pure Yin or pure Yang.

The symbol demonstrates the inter-dependence of Yin and Yang as well. Yin and Yang counterbalance each other, and have within them the natural tendency to bring things back to balance (homoeostasis). We can also see illness in these terms. For example, when we have a high fever, we alternate between periods of sweating and shivering until the fever finally breaks.

THE FIVE ELEMENTS

The concept of the Five Elements or Phases is a further refinement of Yin/Yang. The Five Elements are Water, Wood, Fire, Earth and Metal. Each is associated with a different season, particular emotions and specific organs (see page 24), some of which are different to those we recognise in the West.

Each of the Five Elements is also said to represent a different quality in a person. The Five Elements interact and influence each other. The interactions of the Five Elements are governed by the

THE FIVE ELEMENTS

ELEMENT	SEASON	EMOTION	ORGAN
Wood	Spring	Anger	Liver, Gallbladder
Fire	Summer	Joy	Heart, Small Intestine, Heart Protector, Triple Heater
Earth	Late summer	Pensiveness/ obsessiveness	Spleen, Stomach
Metal	Autumn	Grief	Lungs, Large Intestine
Water	Winter	Fear	Kidney, Bladder

Sheng and Ke cycles. 'Sheng' means 'to promote or engender'. In the Sheng cycle each Element gives birth to the one following it in the circle. So Water produces Wood, Wood produces Fire, Fire produces Earth, Earth produces Metal, and Metal produces Water.

'Ke' means 'control' or 'restraint'. In the Ke cycle each Element controls the next-but-one following it. So Water controls Fire, Wood controls Earth, Fire controls Metal, Earth controls Water, and Metal controls Wood. According to Chinese philosophy, the two cycles must operate together, smoothly and continuously, in order to maintain health. Any imbalance will disturb the whole.

OTHER ELEMENTS

There are other important elements, such as the Six Divisions, the Eight Trigrams, and the Ten Heavenly Stems, but for the purposes of this introduction, the Tao, Yin/Yang and the Five Elements provide the basic building blocks of Traditional Chinese Medicine.

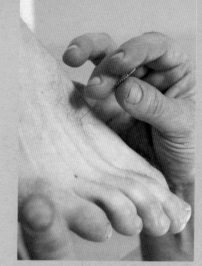

4 How Acupuncture Works

Chinese medicine focuses on five fundamental 'substances' or aspects to a person's being. These are Jing, Qi and Shen (the 'Three Treasures'), Xue ('Blood') and Jin-Ye ('Body Fluids').

JING

This is the deep energy or 'essence' that forms the basic power structure of the body. It determines an individual's, sexual, mental and defensive energies. It is formed from our pre-natal energy, which, according to TCM, determines our constitutional make-up.

QI

Qi is the life force or 'vital energy' of the body. There are different types, associated with different parts of our body, each with its own qualities and functions:

- Original Qi relates to the Kidneys and lower back. It is responsible for the strength of the constitution.
- Defensive Qi relates to the Lungs. It flows on the surface of the body.

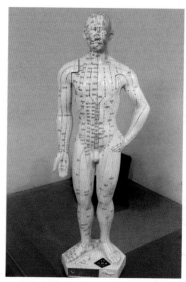

Qi flows in the Jing-Luo (meridian lines), represented on this model.

- Nutritive Qi circulates continuously in the meridians.

When we are healthy, the different types of Qi interact harmoniously, producing a sense of well-being. In illness, specific types of Qi may be deficient or in excess. This produces an imbalance that manifests itself as feelings of ill-health, leading to physical, emotional, psychological or spiritual symptoms.

Qi flows in the Jing-Luo – the invisible network of meridians that integrate the whole energetic functioning of the body (see page 34). Acupuncture works by regulating Qi via needles inserted into points along these meridians. The principle functions of Qi are to:

- **Activate and move:** Life is movement – breathing, eating, walking and so on. Qi governs this movement.
- **Nourish:** Qi nourishes and maintains organs and tissues.
- **Protect:** Qi helps to build up resistance to disease.
- **Warm:** Qi produces warmth through its activity.

SHEN

Shen is the spirit energy. It relates to an individual's attitude, consciousness and mind, and is linked to the Heart.

XUE (BLOOD)

Blood is a dense form of Qi. Its function is to nourish the body. Qi is called the 'commander of the Blood', because of the role it plays in its formation, and because Qi moves Blood around the body. Blood is called the 'mother of Qi', providing nourishment to the body.

JIN-YE (BODY FLUIDS)

Body Fluids moisten and lubricate. There are two types:

- **Jin:** This is thin and watery, and responsible for moistening the skin and hair.
- **Ye:** This is thicker and heavier, and lubricates the joints, sense organs, brain and spinal cord.

It is the balance between the Five Substances that is important. This equilibrium is maintained by the Zang-Fu (the organs). The functions of the Zang-Fu are integrated through the whole body by the meridian network.

ZANG-FU (ORGANS)

The Chinese concept of organs is different from ours. Chinese medicine is more concerned with the organs' function and spheres of influence than with their physical structure. The organs are described either as Zang or Fu (see page 32).

Zang organs

These are the 'solid organs', (see page 32). Zang organs are Yin because they store and preserve important substances, transform and utilise energy, and control the inner workings of the body.

Fu organs

These are the 'hollow organs' (see page 32). The Fu organs are Yang because they are sites of activity and movement, and are involved with the transformation and elimination of impure (waste) substances.

In acupuncture, it is the integrated functioning of all the organs that is important. If one is not working properly, an

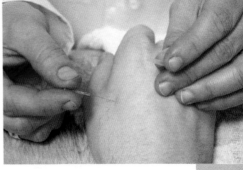

Here the practitioner is needling the acu-point for the Large Intestine, one of the Fu organs.

acupuncturist will explore how this relates to the other organs and treat all affected organs.

All organs, but especially the Zang organs, are responsible for processing and maintenance of Shen, Qi, Jing, Blood and

ORGANS AND THEIR FUNCTIONS

ZANG ORGANS

- **Liver:** Seat of the soul, stores and controls the flow of Qi and Blood around the body.
- **Heart:** Seat of all powers of mind and soul, and controls Blood.
- **Pericardium:** Protects and assists the Heart. (Not strictly an organ, in TCM the Pericardium is 'protector of the Heart', with a strong influence on circulation and sex.)
- **Spleen:** Transforms and transports food, fluids and Qi through the body.
- **Lungs:** Rhythmic regulator, distributes Qi through the body.
- **Kidneys:** Stores Qi, governs growth and development.

FU ORGANS

- **Gall Bladder:** Stores bile, assists Liver.
- **Small Intestine:** Receives and transforms material from Stomach.
- **Triple Heater:** Protector of organs and regulator of temperature and fluid metabolism. (Not strictly an organ, the Triple Heater embraces several complex functions, including distribution of Qi.)
- **Stomach:** Extracts Qi from liquids and solids.
- **Large Intestine:** Absorbs water and nutrients, and eliminates waste as faeces.
- **Bladder:** Accessory to Kidneys, and eliminates waste and urine.

Body Fluids. However, Qi circulates through the meridian pathways, which acupuncturists must 'tap into' in order to stimulate, disperse or redirect the Qi.

JING-LUO (THE MERIDIANS)
Meridians are pathways of energy. TCM describes the meridians according to their positions and functions (see table below).

MERIDIAN POSITIONS AND FUNCTIONS

- **Main meridians (12 pairs):** Directly connected to the organs from which they take their names. They have pathways near the surface and acupuncture points.
- **Extraordinary meridians:** Act as powerful reservoirs for the main meridians. Only two have their own 'points'.
- **'Luo' or Connecting meridians:** Join each main meridian to its paired meridian.
- **Muscle meridians:** Closer to the surface than the main meridians. They nourish muscles and joints.

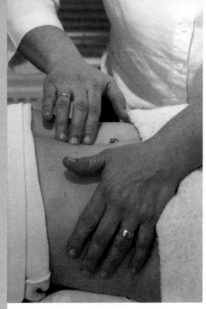

Palpating points on the Ren Mai or 'Conception Vessel'.

The 12 main meridians are bilateral, resulting in 24 separate pathways. Each meridian is related to an organ to which it is connected.

Running vertically up the midline of the body are two 'primary' meridians:

- **Du Mai:** The 'Governing Vessel' that unites the Yang on the back.
- **Ren Mai:** The 'Conception Vessel' that unites the Yin on the front.

All meridians start or end at the hands or feet. Meridians

are also grouped according to the quality of the energy they carry. This produces another six pairs of meridians, each pair made up of one arm and one leg meridian.

Along each meridian there are 'points' that have a particular influence on the Qi. An acupuncturist inserts a needle into a specific point in order to influence the Qi in a particular way.

ILL-HEALTH
Acupuncturists think in terms of the 'depth' of an illness. Put

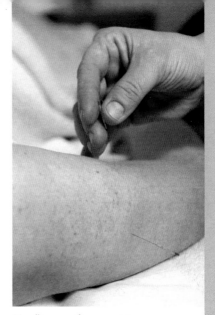

Needling specific acu-points influences the Qi in different ways and restores balance.

simply, 'superficial' illnesses tend to relate to a problem in a particular meridian, whereas more serious ill-health usually relates to the organ itself.

If a superficial illness is not treated, eventually there will be an effect on the organ.

In Chinese medicine, the cause of disease may be congenital, poisons, parasites, accidents, poor diet, exercise or lifestyle.

Causes are also said to be either:

• **External (climatic):** Those that affect the body.

• **Internal (emotional):** Those that affect the mind and the spirit.

The Chinese believe that external causes of disease will affect only those individuals whose Qi is already compromised in some way. External causes include wind, heat, cold, damp, dryness, diet and excess sexual activity (the Chinese are firm believers that too much sex is bad for you). Internal causes relate to the effect on a person's health of extremes or excesses of particular emotions, be it anger, joy, worry or pensiveness, grief, fear or fright.

In all things, practitioners of Chinese medicine advocate the 'middle way', avoiding extremes in order to promote health, happiness and longevity.

BA GANG (THE EIGHT PRINCIPLE PATTERNS)

The Eight Principle Patterns help an acupuncturist to make sense of the signs and symptoms with which a patient presents. In effect, they guide the practitioner towards an accurate diagnosis specific to that person. The patterns are represented as a further differentiation of Yin/Yang:

Yin	Yang
Interior	Exterior
Deficiency	Excess
Cold	Heat

Interior/Exterior

This refers to the depth of a disorder, in terms of its location in the body. Exterior conditions arise from an external cause and are located in the superficial layers of the body. Onset is sudden, affecting the superficial parts of the body and producing chills, fever, headaches or body aches.

Interior conditions are located deeper in the body. They develop gradually. They are chronic, long-term disorders that affect organs, deep tissues or bones. Symptoms include changes in appetite or bowel movements, internal discomfort or pain. They are often reflected in changes to the tongue (see page 53).

Deficiency/Excess

The strength of the body's defences against disease is determined by the pattern of deficiency/excess.

Deficiency shows a general emptiness, and reflects an insufficiency of Blood, Qi or Body Fluids, or the underactivity of an organ. Symptoms include weakness, tiredness, inactivity and a weak voice. There may also be shallow breathing. Pains improve with applied pressure. The pulse is weak (see page 55), and the tongue is pale.

Excess shows either as a

strong reaction to an external attack, or evidence of accumulation and stagnation. Symptoms include heavy and forceful movement, heavy breathing, congestion, fullness, and bloating. The pulse is strong and full.

Cold/Heat

The pattern of Cold/Heat gives clues as to the nature of the disorder. Signs of Cold include a pale complexion, slow movements, a withdrawn manner, wanting to curl up, feeling chilled, lack of thirst or only wanting warm drinks. Pains improve with warmth. Other symptoms include diarrhoea, profuse pale urine, a slow pulse, and a pale and swollen tongue coved with what looks like white fur.

Signs of Heat include a red face, fever, dislike of warmth, irritability, thirst, constipation, scant dark urine, red skin eruptions, fast pulse, and a red tongue with yellow fur.

DIAGNOSIS

Using the principles and patterns of Chinese medicine,

an acupuncturist can draw up an intricate and specific picture of each patient's problems. With a very precise and detailed diagnosis, acupuncture is then used to restore balance, resulting in disappearance of the symptoms.

FIVE ELEMENT ACUPUNCTURE

According to TCM, close observation of the Elements around us (Water, Wood, Earth, Fire and Metal) has led to the belief that we are microcosms of the macrocosm – we are intricately linked with, and affected by, the world around us.

Every individual reflects all aspects of life. For example, the renewed drive to make changes in the spring. However, each of us tends to reflect one element to a greater degree than the rest, which has a subtle influence on the way we interpret and behave in the world.

For example, if you are a Wood type, you may really like (or sometimes dislike) the spring. You may feel particularly alive and well at this time or possibly out of sorts. Just as a tall tree needs both flexibility and firmness in the face of a strong wind, you may have issues around uprightness or rigidity. A need to speak out and be forthright (or contrastingly an inability to take courage) may also be indicative of 'Woody' energy.

A practitioner using the Law of the Five Elements will identify a patient's Element or constitutional type through closely observing colour, sound, odour and emotion (see Chapter Six). This becomes part of the detailed diagnosis that the practitioner makes, together with all the other signs and symptoms of illness, and helps to determine the best treatment for that particular patient.

JAPANESE ACUPUNCTURE
Japanese acupuncture traditions are based on the same Chinese medical texts. However, where TCM emphasises the organ systems, Japanese acupuncture

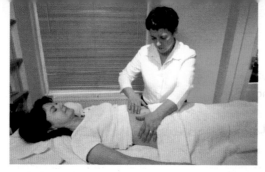

Abdominal diagnosis is a very important tool in Japanese acupuncture.

(meridian therapy, in particular) emphasises the balance of the Qi flowing in the channels.

Once acupuncture reached Japan, the Japanese developed and refined their own techniques. For example, the 'shinkan' guide tube was developed in the late 1600s by a blind practitioner to enable easier insertion of needles. This is still pertinent today, as some 40 per cent of Japanese practitioners are blind. Today, guide tubes are extensively used by practitioners of all styles of acupuncture.

The long-standing tradition of Japanese blind practitioners

explains why touch plays such a major part in Japanese acupuncture diagnosis.

SCIENTIFIC EXPLANATIONS

Western science's attempts to explain how acupuncture works tend to fall into one of three popular types of explanation:

- That the nerve fibres carry and transmit the acupuncture effect.
- That the circulation of neurotransmitters and other hormones (particularly endorphins) in the blood and cerebrospinal fluid causes the effect.
- That the meridians are electrically distinct, and that changes within them are responsible for triggering neural and humoral (bodily fluids) responses.

However, despite the undeniable success rate of acupuncture, there remains, to date, no Western scientific theory that has proved wholly satisfactory in explaining how acupuncture achieves such results.

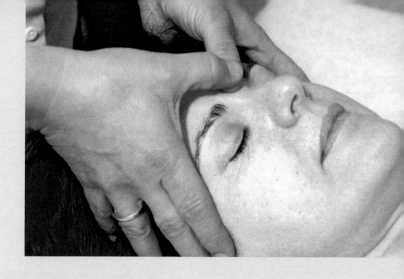

5 Will Acupuncture Work For Me?

Chinese medicine has traditionally been used to maintain health, and acupuncture appointments were booked rather like a car service – at regular intervals.

In the West however, most people tend to experience their first session in an attempt to overcome a specific problem.

DISEASE

The World Health Organisation endorses the use of acupuncture for certain conditions (see pages 6 to 7).

In both China and the West, acupuncture has been used to treat almost the entire spectrum of illness – physical and psychological, acute and chronic.

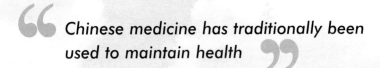

Chinese medicine has traditionally been used to maintain health

❶ PREVENTATIVE HEALTH CARE

Chang is 49, the second generation of a Hong Kong Chinese family who settled in the UK in the 1950s. He has always used TCM.

"In our culture you go for a treatment at the change of the season, to help you make the transition smoothly. I always find it very relaxing, and afterwards I feel invigorated. If I do get sick, my first action is to call up my acupuncturist. He knows me very well by now, and knows my weak areas. The treatments are always successful. I think, because I use acupuncture regularly, any health problem I get is only very 'superficial' in Chinese terms, and is quickly and easily dealt with."

❷ IRRITABLE BOWEL SYNDROME

Amy is 36, married and working full-time. She visited her GP with symptoms that turned out to be irritable bowel syndrome (IBS). Her GP linked the condition with stress and suggested a course with the acupuncturist practising at the surgery.

Amy had 10 sessions, after which her stress and IBS were under control. Her practitioner also suggested some lifestyle and dietary changes and, says Amy, "I did everything she said – I didn't want to be a victim of IBS! And guess what – now I'm pregnant too, something I didn't think would be possible."

When asked if acupuncture hurt, Amy says, "I was made to breathe deeply and my acupuncturist put the needles in as I exhaled. Only the odd needle actually hurt."

Between treatments, Amy wore special studs on her inner ear lobe, and her acupuncturist also used the burning herb moxa (see page 59) to support the treatments she gave Amy. "I found the theory behind acupuncture made sense – the idea of relieving pressure points and getting energy or Qi to flow. It tied in with my feelings of being stuck," concludes Amy.

3 RENAL PAIN

Jennifer was 23 when she collapsed with an acute kidney infection – pyelonephritis.

Treated with conventional medicine, Jennifer recovered. However, she continued to experience a constant dull ache in her lower back around the area of her right kidney, which sometimes flared up into full-blown renal colic.

Apart from offering painkillers, her doctor was unable to help. Eventually, a friend took the reluctant Jennifer to an acupuncturist.

Jennifer recalls: "Almost as soon as the needles were all in, I felt the pain drain away – it was like a miracle. Basically, the acupuncturist said that while the infection had gone, my whole system was still unbalanced and a product of the imbalance was the pain I was getting. I went back two more times and then I was officially declared well. That was three years ago and the pain has never returned."

Gavin is in his 40s and originally went to an acupuncturist for chronic sinusitis.

However, Gavin also suffers from regular epileptic attacks, something that started when he was a child. The attacks were trigged by stimulation or excitement. Gavin has taken conventional medication for his epilepsy for many years, and the condition seemed to be largely under control.

His acupuncturist explains the treatment he gave Gavin:

"I found that Gavin's Kidney and Liver Yin were weak, which allowed the Liver Wind to develop inside when the Liver energy was stimulated too strongly. In Chinese medicine this means the Liver Wind stirs up excess Phlegm, which moves upwards, clouding the mind and confusing the senses – leading to an epileptic attack. I gave Gavin a treatment to clear the Phlegm and to calm the Liver by strengthening the Kidneys and drawing excess Qi down from the head."

Gavin's sinus problem cleared quite quickly, but as a result of regular acupuncture treatments over the subsequent year, he has been able to reduce his epilepsy medication, and the fits.he has experienced have been much less frequent and less severe.

❺ SMOKING ADDICTION

Adam had been a smoker for nearly a decade, but when he turned 30, he decided to stop.

Attempts at 'cold turkey' and nicotine patches failed, so his girlfriend suggested hypnosis or acupuncture. Adam decided that "having needles stuck in me was a lesser evil to handing my mind over to some therapist."

At his first appointment, the acupuncturist found that Adam's energy was low and out of balance. She suggested a few treatments to 'harmonise Adam's Qi' before he tried to give up smoking. Reluctantly Adam agreed, but says, "In actual fact, after three treatments I felt so much more healthy and relaxed, giving up smoking just didn't seem such a problem. In the first few weeks after giving up, I went back for some support treatments, but after that, I stopped wanting a ciggie and took up badminton instead!"

❺ INSOMNIA

Maureen is in her late 50s and has insomnia. She had been taking sleeping tablets for six months, but they were losing their effect. Reluctant to increase her dose, Maureen decided to try acupuncture.

Her acupuncturist says: "Maureen also has migraine headaches. I diagnosed excess Liver Fire affecting the spirit, so I aimed to balance the Liver function, calm the nerves and quieten the Spirit."

After six treatments, Maureen was sleeping without the help of drugs and she was also migraine-free.

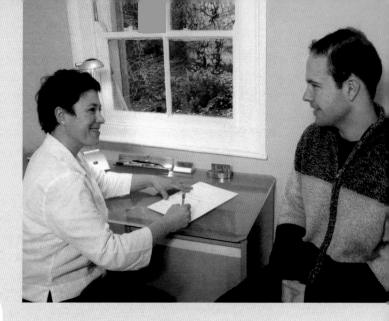

6 What To Expect

A first appointment with an acupuncturist normally lasts up to an hour and a half. This is because the practitioner needs to spend more time making an initial diagnosis.

LOOKING

Your acupuncturist will note the way you walk in and sit down, your facial expressions, responses, and general bearing throughout the consultation (see picture on left). These observations help to assess your 'spirit' (Shen).

The acupuncturist will also examine your facial colour. All the meridians flow to the face, so the state of Blood and Qi is evident in your colouring.

TONGUE DIAGNOSIS

The tongue's shape, colour, coating and texture provide vital information on the state of the organs.

A healthy tongue should be reddish with little or no fur. It should not be swollen or contracted, or have cracks on the surface or teeth marks along the edge. If you eat or

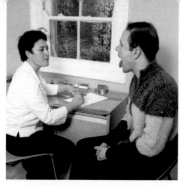

Tongue diagnosis is an important part of acupuncture.

drink just before your appointment, this can give a misleading picture.

LISTENING AND SMELLING
The sound of your voice and your breathing are also helpful indicators. A loud, assertive voice, for example, suggests a Yang pattern, whereas a weak, timid voice suggests Yin.

'Smelling' is a bit of a no-no in Western etiquette, but traditionally, body smells are considered important.

ASKING
During your first consultation you will be asked a range of questions about your physical, emotional and energy state. Some may seem unrelated to your problem, but your acupuncturist will ask these

questions to form a complete picture of your condition.

You will also have to give a full medical history, which may also include that of your family.

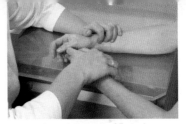
Your balance of energy can be assessed from the pulse.

TOUCHING

In some styles of acupuncture, particularly Japanese, abdominal palpation is another major diagnostic tool. The main organs are represented on the abdomen, which provides valuable information about their condition.

The abdomen, like the pulse, changes during the treatment session, often instantaneously. It is a helpful indicator of how you are responding to treatment.

THE PULSE

Taking the pulse is one of the fundamental diagnostic tools of TCM. It is important that you are relaxed for this, so if you were late or in a hurry when you arrived, you may be asked to lie for a few minutes to allow the pulse to settle.

An acupuncturist will assess your balance of energy from three positions in the wrist of each hand that correspond to the upper, middle and lower areas of the body. The depth, speed, general quality and overall balance of the pulses give information on your internal state.

The qualities of the pulse can be divided into those relating to Yin and those to Yang:

Yin	Yang
Slow	Fast
Deep	Superficial
Choppy	Slippery
Empty	Full

BEFORE YOU GO
It is best to avoid some things immediately before and directly after an acupuncture treatment because they are thought to affect your Qi – this can counteract the effect of treatment. These include:
- Alcohol
- Excessive fatigue and hunger

- Large meals
- Sexual activity
- Hot baths
- Extreme emotional states.

RECEIVING TREATMENT

Once an acupuncturist has made a diagnosis, the next step is to plan the treatment. This involves selecting specific acupuncture points, massage, and possibly the use of moxibustion (see page 59). You may also be prescribed herbs, and most practitioners give suggestions about diet and exercise.

NEEDLES

Acupuncturists generally use very fine, single-use disposable needles made of stainless steel. All acupuncturists registered with a professional body will be required to observe stringent standards of hygiene and sterilization for needles and other equipment.

Most people receiving acupuncture for the first time are concerned that it will hurt. While it should not be painful when the needles are inserted, there is a 'needle sensation' that may be a tingling or feeling of numbness. There may also be a stronger sensation when the needle comes into contact with Qi that lasts for a second or two. This is called De Qi, and indicates that the Qi is responding.

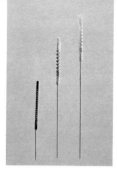

Acupuncture needles are made of stainless steel, and acupuncturists observe strict standards of hygiene.

Different styles of acupuncture insert needles to varying depths. For example, in Japanese acupuncture, extremely fine needles are usually inserted very superficially and the De Qi sensation is not felt.

The choice of acupuncture points will be specific to your needs, and the needles are left in for varying lengths of time, usually around 10-20 minutes, although sometimes the practitioner may insert a needle and then withdraw it almost immediately, as may be the case with the treatment of children. Additionally, there are many techniques specific to children that do not involve inserting needles. These techniques can be taught to parents who can reinforce treatment at home.

MONITORING

You will normally be asked to lie down during treatment, and your acupuncturist may take your pulse at intervals. After removing the needles, your pulses will be taken again, as a measure of the success of the treatment.

MOXIBUSTION

Moxa comes from the dried leaves of the common mugwort (*Artemisia vulgaris*). Small balls may be placed on the end of acupuncture needles and burned gently, or small cones can be placed directly on the skin to smoulder (they are removed long before they cause any discomfort or pain). Also, a cigar-shaped roll can be lit at one end and moved slowly over the skin and particular acu-points. Moxa heats the Qi gently and helps tonification (a method of stimulating Qi used when Qi is thought to be weak). It can be a very pleasant and relaxing experience. You may be given such a moxa stick to use at home in between treatments.

CUPPING

Cupping is another useful adjunct technique. It is used for to treat stagnation and cold.

A vacuum is created inside a glass or bamboo cup by briefly inserting a flame and then placing the cup on the skin, or by using cups that have a suction pump.

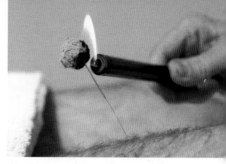

Moxibustion enhances the toning effect of acupuncture.

POST TREATMENT

After your treatment you may be offered advice on your lifestyle (to support the effects of the treatment). You will also be told whether further treatment is needed and how long for.

Finding a practitioner

TRADITIONAL

Traditional acupuncturists practise according to the philosophical principles of TCM, and are trained in the Western medical sciences appropriate to the practice of acupuncture. Contact:

The British Acupuncture Council

63 Jeddo Road,
London, W12 9HQ.
Tel: 020 8735 0400
Website:
www.acupuncture.org.uk
Email:
info@acupuncture.org.uk

MEDICAL

Doctors who undertake a training course can use acupuncture within their practice, but they may not practise using TCM principles. Contact:

The British Medical Acupuncture Society (BMAS)

12 Marbury House,
High Whitley, Cheshire,
Warrington, WA4 4QW.
Tel: 01925 730727
Website: www.medical-
acupuncture.co.uk
Email: admin@medical-
acupuncture.org.uk

About the author

Joanna Trevelyan is an experienced writer and journalist with a particular interest in complementary therapies, health and nursing, environmental health issues, alternative lifestyles, and women's issues. She has written for a wide range of professional bodies, including the World Health Organisation, the Natural Medicines Society, the Parliamentary Group for Complementary and Alternative Medicine, and the foundation for Integrated Health. Joanna has also been editor of the professional journal *Nursing Times*. In 1994, she was awarded a Commendation in the Medical Journalism Awards.

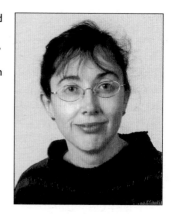

ACKNOWLEDGEMENTS
Special thanks are due to The British Acupuncture Council for help with photography, and also to practitioner Marian Fixler, who is portrayed in the photographs.

Other titles in the series

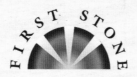

First published in 2004 by First Stone Publishing
PO Box 8, Lydney, Gloucestershire, GL15 6YD

The contents of this book are for information only and are not intended as a substitute for appropriate medical attention. The author and publishers admit no liability for any consequences arising from following any advice contained within this book. If you have any concerns about your health or medication, always consult your doctor.

ISBN 1 904439 26 8

Printed and bound in Hong Kong through Sino Publishing House Ltd.